# Health improvement through Body Knowledge

A. Gabriel

Published by Angel E Mendez, 2024.

HEALTH IMPROVEMENT THROUGH BODY KNOWLEDGE

**First edition. February 3, 2024.**

Copyright © 2024 A. Gabriel.

ISBN: 979-8224009718

Written by A. Gabriel.

# Health improvement through Body Knowledge

Healthy and Longevity Fit
By A Gabriel

# Introduction

In the early 1980s, a Japanese Forest Agency started advising people to take regular walks in the woods to maintain good health. Although, even today, not all people take this advice seriously, walking or jogging under the sun's rays can be medicinal, especially for those experiencing muscle aches or related illnesses. Sometimes this referred practice of forest bathing can lower stress and alleviate body aches.

However, evidence shows that spending time in nature leads to healthy changes and other bodily benefits.

Therapy experts in Orient countries have discovered that walking for at least forty minutes in cedar forests can help reduce cortisol levels, a stress hormone linked to blood pressure and immune system functions.

However, walking for the same duration in a lab did not yield the same physiological relaxation effects as walking in a forest.

According to Japanese research, trees, and plants release aromatic compounds known as phytoncides.

And inhaling these compounds can provide therapeutic benefits.

Like those of aromatherapy, sleeping in a forest can also improve blood protection against diseases like cancer, boost immunity, and lowers blood pressure.

The body can experience positive effects from being in a beautiful forest environment with the fresh scent of nature and clean air.

The great news is that visiting green spaces is affordable for enhancing health.

Other recent studies have shown that almost ten percent of people with high blood pressure managed it by walking for thirty minutes or relaxing in a park or other green areas.

Among the advantages of being in a forest is the fresh air.

Studies show that people living in cities with more polluted air have a higher risk of heart attacks.

However, other factors can contribute to the risk of illnesses in city dwellers.

Being exposed to beautiful environments like waterfalls or peaceful countryside can positively impact the body and mind.

Such pleasant views can evoke awe and thankfulness, which benefit the mind.

In 2015, a researcher from the University of California discovered that individuals who could appreciate the magnificence of tall trees were generally kinder to others than those who could not notice anything extraordinary in regular trees.

Meditation cultivates a mindset open to appreciating the world's wonders beyond oneself, promoting a sense of selflessness, and enhancing overall well-being, including physical health.

Residing in cities with large green areas can enhance energy levels, promote well-being, and elevate mood and happiness.

A 2016 study showed that women residing in areas with abundant vegetation had a 12% lower risk of diseases than those living in densely populated urban areas.

Breathing in the fresh air of nature can have medicinal benefits. Walking through a forest, for example, allows you to inhale phytoncides ( Phytoncides are antimicrobial allelochemical volatile organic compounds derived from plants) which can boost natural killer cells (NK), a type of white blood cell that strengthens the immune system and therefore lower the risk of developing health issues such as cancer, heart disease, and diabetes.

Additionally, a study discovered that being in a room with those same phytoncides, often found in forests, to a certain degree, can have the same benefits as walking or inhaling those antimicrobial allelochemical compounds derived from plants.

Unsurprisingly, those residing in urban areas tend to experience more anxiety and aggression compared to those in rural and less populated areas.

Unfortunately, more people live in cities than in rural regions.

As a result, studies generally indicate that individuals living close to or in natural surroundings have better physical and mental health.

Researchers have yet to determine the precise method by which nature improves mood disorders in humans.

However, studies suggest that the air near rivers, forests, and mountains contains molecules charged with electricity and sun rays that may help alleviate symptoms of depression, as reported by Frontiers in Psychology.

Another observation reveals that children with ADHD may experience improved behavior and attention when walking in nature compared to urban areas.

Therefore, spending time in a relaxing natural environment promotes well-being.

Fortunately, interacting with natural environments can improve attention and concentration for most people.

Even those with short-term memory issues can experience a 20% boost in memory by taking walks in forests or parks.

Studies have proven that having plants in a room or house can positively impact people's well-being.

Even the simple act of viewing trees from a window can offer a range of benefits.

Additionally, even artificial nature in the form of images, sounds, or smells can positively affect individuals.

Moreover, listening to sounds through headphones has been shown to assist patients in recovering faster from stress and other illnesses.

Research has confirmed that people who spend time in nature can benefit from improved attention, reduced stress levels, and faster recovery from illnesses.

And in some cases, people with more contact with nature require less medication while recovering.

The publisher owns the rights to this work. Therefore, this work's partial or total reproduction by any means electronic or mechanical, including photocopying, recording, or by any information storage and retrieval system or method without the publisher's written authorization is prohibited.

# Chapter One

# Benefits of barefoot walking

"There's nothing in the mechanical world that matches the sophistication, complexity, and multi-tasking ability of the foot."

— Michael Sandler, Barefoot Running

Perhaps you have experienced walking barefoot and felt an incredible sensation.

This sensation is because the earth is full of potent energy, and when your bare feet contact the ground, your body absorbs the earth's electrons.

This earth energy is unique and can nourish both your body and mind.

Some refer to this healing experience as Earthing.

Did you know that earthing has numerous health benefits that can improve your daily life, including enhancing your eyesight? According to a study called reflexology or zone therapy, certain areas on the feet connect to the eye nerve system.

By applying pressure to these areas on the feet, you can energize your eyesight and relax the muscles related to the eyes.

This alternative medical practice also involves applying pressure to other body parts, such as the ears and hands, using thumb fingers and massage techniques without using oils or lotions.

Research shows that walking barefoot can also calm the mind, reducing stress by up to 60 percent due to the increased production of endorphins or "feel good" hormones.

Walking without shoes can help stretch and relax the feet muscles, ligaments, and tendons.

It also strengthens the flexors, reducing pain for those with flat feet.

Walking barefoot on grass has several health benefits.

It can help stabilize your circadian rhythm, leading to better sleep and balanced hormones.

Additionally, it can promote cardiovascular health by improving the balance of your autonomic nervous system.

Walking barefoot can also benefit blood viscosity, boost brain power, and improve heart rate.

Connecting with the Earth through your feet can boost your body's antioxidants, lower inflammation, and enhance sleep quality.

Research indicates that grounding barefoot for only 30 minutes can improve a variety of bodily ailments.

However, if someone has diabetes, they may experience complications if they get a cut or injury on their foot while walking without shoes.

Walking barefoot in woods or forests can be risky due to poisonous insects like ants and other small animals.

So always be cautious.

Throughout history, humans and animals have relied on their close relationship with nature to survive and thrive.

However, in modern times, many people have lost touch with nature due to their lifestyle choices.

We now sleep on beds, wear shoes to walk and run, travel by cars and planes, and observe forests from a distance.

And unfortunately, this disconnection from nature has been linked to physiological dysfunction and poorer health, despite our reluctance to admit it.

Spending time in nature and connecting with the earth can have several benefits, such as feeling refreshed, motivated, and in sync with nature.

Engaging in mindfulness while being in nature can provide a feeling of calmness and enjoyment and increase our awareness and alertness.

The soil is home to microbes, and exposure to it can naturally boost the human body's immune system.

Though there is a belief that walking barefoot increases the risk of a cold or cough, this is not entirely true, as catching a cold is influenced by various natural factors and one's immune system.

Besides, diverse cultures frequently walk barefoot and traditionally do not experience an unusually high rate of colds.

Orthopedic professionals agree that the padding and structure of shoes can prevent people's feet from using specific groups of ligaments and muscles related to the body.

Also, walking barefoot can help restore a natural posture, improve balance, alleviate knee pain, and restore correct hip mechanics.

Numerous studies on barefoot walking have shown several health benefits.

Still, only some people benefit from them due to a lack of contact with the earth's grass and soil and because of today's people's lifestyle.

The human body is bioelectrical, with a slight positive charge, and conducts electrical impulses that allow the brain to function and send signals.

The resting cells charge negatively internally, and the overall charge in the body is positive due to a slight imbalance of ions.

If the feet make physical contact with the negatively charged earth, the excess energy in the body discharges, resulting in a healing effect at the cellular level.

Resting cells do not undergo division, have reduced or absent endogenous respiration, and naturally form a resting stage as part of their life cycle.

So, for natural healing, walking barefoot on grass, dirt, or sand is the easiest way to well-being.

Studies have shown that inflammation is the leading cause of chronic pain and several significant health conditions, including cardiovascular disease, diabetes, and certain types of cancer.

Inflammation is the immune system's natural response to intruding viruses, bacteria, and foreign substances like pollen and air pollutants.

While inflammation is necessary to combat common colds and allergies, persistent inflammation can harm healthy cells.

Walking barefoot on the ground can improve our immunity by reducing white blood cells and increasing red blood cells.

This practice also increases antioxidants, reduces inflammation, and improves sleep.

Additionally, other alternative ways of grounding involve direct or indirect contact with the earth's healing properties.

Although further research is needed to understand the benefits of barefoot walking fully, many health professionals acknowledge that feeling connected to nature is a significant advantage.

Fortunately, there is no harm in experiencing this connection.

Barefoot walking is a simple therapeutic technique done in nature, and it is available to anyone for at least three seasons of the year.

Remove your shoes and enjoy walking on the grass to promote a healthy lifestyle.

Runners who have tried this approach believe it works well, though this running style may require some precautions.

Barefoot running is nothing new; however, many runners have discovered the advantages of running barefoot in recent years.

Among the advantages of barefoot running is that it can help to build and develop the muscles of the feet to prevent injuries.

This assertion does not mean one should ditch shoes, but instead, barefoot running can be seen as a training tool.

It's noteworthy and important to note that humans didn't always have cushioned soles or arch supports.

In some places, people have run with only their skin touching the ground.

However, the recommendation is to look for the advice of a good sports physical therapist before trying this running style.

It is essential to recognize the significance of the 1960 Tokyo Marathon, particularly the remarkable achievement of Ethiopian runner Abebe Bikila.

Despite having new running shoes for the Rome Olympics, Bikila found them too small, and they caused painful blisters. As a result, he chose to run the entire 42,195 m race barefoot.

This decision made history; he won the race and set a world record for the distance, timing 2 hours, 15 minutes, and 16.2 seconds.

Bikila was also the first African to win an Olympic medal, breaking his record four years later, securing his second Olympic gold title.

Advancements in running shoe technology have progressed in the past century.

Today's shoe features include arch support, ridged soles to minimize shin splints, and, most recently, carbon-fiber plates between the shoe's midsole, making it ultra-lightweight and energy-returning.

These innovations are intended to help athletes perform their best, helping to lead to world records, especially in the marathon. However, it is not all about footwear.

Abebe Bikila, who won an Olympic gold medal, ran barefoot because his shoes fell apart just days before the race.

Still, usually, Bikila used to train without shoes suitable for his feet.

The question is.

Is running barefoot good for you?

Research does not give a conclusive answer on the advantages of barefoot running.

However, runners out there are increasing trends of "natural running," with many believing that running without shoes decreases the likelihood of long-term injuries because of a better running technique, leading to greater efficiency in movement or mechanics.

A barefoot running style results in shorter strides.

And the strides go more centered beneath your torso and better align with your body's center of gravity.

This type of gait often results in a more significant bend in the knee, allowing your joints to absorb the shock of impact better.

Barefoot runners typically land more on the ball of their foot than the heel, improving movement efficiency.

And natural running patterns can reduce joint loading, making it a healthy choice for runners.

Other benefits of barefoot running are the strengthening and tightening foot muscles that stabilize a flat arch.

Wearing supportive shoes all the time can prevent the building of muscular strength in your feet to support bones that may naturally be less tight in structure.

However, if running barefoot causes you pain or discomfort, it's best to wear shoes or start practicing barefoot running more gradually.

Running without shoes may reduce the risk of plantar fasciitis while improving technique and cadence.

A poor running technique can lead to strain in your lower leg muscles.

In addition, running without shoes leads to increased calorie burn.

However, concerns exist about the potential discomfort and injury risks associated with running barefoot, such as stepping on rocks, sticks, prickly weeds, and even poisonous insects.

Running without shoes exposes the feet to cuts, puncture wounds, and, therefore, to infections. Besides, running barefoot on hot pavement or in extreme cold inevitably harms the soles of your feet.

It's not surprising that running barefoot can lead to an increased risk of foot stress fractures.

It is important to note that people with diabetic conditions may experience severe foot problems, so running barefoot may not be the best idea. Ultimately, it's up to the runner or walker to consider their health condition and the surface they're running on when deciding whether to run barefoot.

So, the best way to incorporate barefoot running or training into your fitness routine is to treat it as a supplement to your regular practice on safe surfaces.

Still, barefoot running is a good training component.

This way, you can safely use barefoot running as a complementary tool to enhance your running or walking performance.

And there are different types of running shoes available in the market.

Some sports shoes offer less cushioning and support than average running shoes but still provide a certain level of protection for your feet.

When trying barefoot running, the best is to take it slow and transition gradually.

The best way is to start by planning how to give your feet and the leg muscles time to adapt.

Start by wearing less cushioned shoes with little drops from heel to toe.

To help your body adjust to minimalist shoes, cut your weekly mileage in half, and gradually increase your distance each week based on your comfort level.

Practicing barefoot running and walking will strain some muscles more than others, as well as the joints and tendons.

A helpful method for efficient muscle recovery after transitioning from running shoes to barefoot running is to massage the lower legs and feet meridians.

Individuals who opt for barefoot running may experience different levels of adaptation.

So, starting with softer surfaces when attempting shorter distances is advisable until one's feet feel accustomed to running without shoes.

Gradually increasing the distance is the recommended approach for barefoot running.

Whether someone decides to run or walk, with or without shoes, it is crucial to maintain a comfortable form when performing this physical activity.

Running barefoot can improve muscle health, enhance foot and leg performance, restore natural form, and improve technique.

But before starting a walking or running exercise routine barefoot, it is necessary to undergo a medical examination to ensure optimal physical health.

# Chapter Two

# Biofield

"I go to nature to be soothed, healed and have my senses put in order."

– John Burroughs

The field of medicine is evolving, and the focus has shifted from simply treating illnesses to promoting overall health and wellness.

This approach combines traditional and modern methods to provide more comprehensive patient care.

This new model recognizes the complexity of our biology and acknowledges that addressing the root cause of specific health issues requires looking beyond traditional molecular approaches.

Advancements in biophysics, biology, psychology, and mind-body research have contributed to the development of this integrative medical model. Examples include psychoneuroimmunology and psychosocial genomics, which have paved the way for this expanded approach to healthcare.

Living systems respond to energy fields alongside biochemical signals for physiological regulation.

Different sources influence this concept, including complementary and alternative medicine therapies and Western biomedicine's use of electrocardiograms and electroencephalograms.

Cell biology and biophysics research also suggests that electromagnetic and other fields contribute to development, tissue repair, and other hemodynamic processes.

So, the biofield is an idea that bridges traditional and modern explanations for energy medicine on how living systems maintain balance.

Through it, we can gain insight into biology and energy medicine, which involves applying low-level signals to the body for healing.

Though not well understood by the traditional biomedical approach, which focuses on chemistry and drugs.

The biofield is a complex energy field that regulates biological processes, and it provides a valuable foundation for energy medicine research and practice.

Throughout history, two opposing views have been on the nature of life.

Democritus, who coined the term "atom," believed everything, including living organisms, could be broken down into constituent parts.

In contrast, Aristotle believed that life processes were self-contained and that all organisms were complete entities.

These two perspectives are molecular reductionism and a holistic view of life.

Practitioners of contemporary complementary medicine use descriptive terms like Chinese qi, Japanese ki, and other similar words to detect imbalances and regulate energy flow to promote healing.

Other alternative medicines have a base on the principle of a vital force.

Chiropractic, homeopathic, and osteopathy practices aim to restore that life force to promote well-being and healing.

The idea of force is a critical concept in physics, while the view of vital force that underlies many CAM therapies is a metaphysical concept by mainstream science.

Force, field, and energy are fundamental concepts in physical theory.

Modern physics recognizes types of force in nature: gravity, electromagnetism, and nuclear forces.

Each force is associated with a particular form of energy, such as electric, magnetic, and electromagnetic, which are particularly important in living systems.

The concept of the biofield is scientifically grounded, although other potential fields could also be involved.

The idea of a biological field introduced in embryology is a way to explain the process of development.

Scientists have discovered many instances of bioelectromagnetic activities that are associated with energies below thermal noise levels.

These activities significantly affect growth, wound repair, regeneration, pain, and decreasing inflammation.

Additionally, field-like phenomena are a link to the principles of biological organization, including embryonic development and the maintenance of physical structure and function. Studies have shown that EMFs can even contribute to the regenerative healing of limbs in animals like salamanders and higher animals.

Furthermore, patterning cell membrane resting potentials is crucial in directing stem cell behavior during embryogenesis and complex organ regeneration.

The Biofield concept research involves practitioners working directly with patients, animals, or cell cultures, which include hands-on therapy, therapeutic touch, and healing touch.

The physical effects of touch on biofield interactions and outcomes are continually studied.

Nonlocal biofield therapies suggest that physical touch may not be the only factor.

Some experts have proposed explanations involving quantum entanglement or other nonlocal causes.

Biofield or Bioenergetics is a biochemistry and cell biology field that concerns energy flow through living systems.

This energy surrounds the body and can extend up to 8 feet from it.

Although invisible to the human eye, people can sense this energy through contact or pressure from some people's hands.

Johrei, which means "purification of the spirit," is a Japanese healing technique developed by Mokichi Okada in the 1930s.

The technique involves directing healing energy towards patients by holding the palms of the hands towards the body and is a basic form of biofield therapy.

Although the exact mechanisms of Johrei healing are poorly understood, Kenji Yamamoto, a professor Emeritus at Kyushu University, has conducted a series of controlled experiments to determine its efficacy.

Biofield therapy does not require any invasion during which the practitioner works with the energy fields of the recipient to promote healing.

This technique improves the recipient's mental and physical well-being and enhances their natural healing power.

The therapist refrains from any physical touch with the patient, instead focusing on projecting positive energy and visualizing it into the patient's body, intending to promote their well-being and happiness.

Okada's concept suggests that every living being has a physical body in the natural world and a spiritual body in the spiritual world.

By cleansing the spiritual body, one can achieve harmony between the body and mind, eliminate negative energy, and alleviate suffering.

However, the practice of Johrei is limited to a few countries due to limited evidence of its effectiveness as a healing therapy and a need for more understanding about it.

Research conducted on Johrei through in vitro studies has demonstrated that the therapy's effectiveness is not limited to attacking cancerous cells but also includes positive effects on the body's healthy cells.

The results of in vitro experiments indicate that Johrei may discourage the growth of abnormal/cancerous cells and promote the development of normal/healthy cells.

However, further testing on patients is necessary to confirm these effects and evaluate their impact.

Previous studies of Johrei suggest a relationship between the enhancement of the immune system and positive effects on mood and stress.

Yamamoto's study has provided remarkable evidence that Johrei therapy can improve blood flow and increase body temperature in people who are generally healthy or those who tend to hypothermia.

However, it is essential to note that only a qualified practitioner should administer the therapy.

Additionally, Yamamoto suggests that Johrei therapy has natural healing properties that may help maintain the body's equilibrium or homeostasis.

The tendency towards maintaining a relatively stable state between elements by physiological processes is called homeostasis.

# Chapter 3

# Solfeggio frequencies

Sound is one of the purest forms of energy in existence.

-Unknown

In the Holy Bible, we find a story about how certain music can benefit an overwhelmed person's mind and spirit due to frustration and stress.

According to the book of 1 Samuel, chapter 16, when the king's servants saw Saul's torment, they said, "Behold now, an evil spirit from God is tormenting you.

Tell our lord, therefore, to your servants who are before you that they seek out someone who knows how to play the harp so that when the evil spirit from God comes upon you, he will play with his hand, and you will be relieved."

So, one of the king's servants recommended David to him, describing him, among other things, as a great harp player. Saul called David and found great consolation in him:

"And when David came to Saul, he stood before him, loved him very much, and made him his armor bearer.

And Saul sent to Jesse, saying, I beg you, David be with me, for he has found favor in my sight."

And when the evil spirit from God came upon Saul, David took the harp and played with his hand; Saul was relieved and was better, and the evil spirit departed from him.

So, the indications are music is powerful and has healing properties.

And we can study something about those healing properties,

including Solfeggio frequencies which are a set of 9 electromagnetic tones that are reputed to have the power to heal and raise consciousness.

Solfeggio frequencies comprise a 6-tone from the music scale, widely used in the 10th century for religious music.

These six tones are known to have healing properties that promote well-being.

As mentioned, these healing music frequencies have existed since early Biblical times.

The Solfeggio frequencies are mainly associated with the Gregorian Chants, a monophonic style used in the Catholic church that dates to the 9th and 10th centuries.

(Hz) Hertz's measurement of solfeggio frequencies and them

Healing benefits follow this order.

396 Hz: is thought to help liberate us from guilt and fear, arguably one of the biggest obstacles we face in life.

417 Hz: helps undo situations and facilitates change in our lives.

It alleviates the conscious and subconscious mind from past traumatic experiences.

528 Hz: the most famous of the frequencies because of its reputation for creat profound transformations and miracles.

It has links to human DNA and the building blocks of our bodies and minds.

639 Hz: is said to improve connection and relationships with people around us, including healing strained relationships and creating new ones.

741 Hz: connected to expression, it helps open our gifts to the world.

852 Hz: finally, one of the original notes returns us to the spiritual and sublime.

An example of the scale on the Hymn to St. John the Baptist, in Latin, Ut queant laxis, is an 8th-century poem attributed to a monk named Paulus Diaconus.

Here is the first poem's stanza:

Ut queant laxis

Resonare fibris

Mira gestorum

Famuli tuorum

Solve polluti

labii reatum

Sancte Johannes.

The first syllable lines-Ut-Re-Mi-Fa-Sol-La is the basis for the Do-Re-Mi-Fa-So-La-Ti, the same scale used today but adding another note to the original six-tone Solfege.

There's musical, historical, and religious importance involved.

But these frequencies also have healing attributes.

However, it has also been hard for some people to believe or easy to be dismissive when first introduced to the Solfeggio frequencies and their purported benefits.

But for a long time, many people have believed in music's healing properties, and scientific research indicates that these solfeggio frequencies are truly healing.

On the other hand, the therapeutic value of music has had recognition since ancient times.

Physicians from the past have used musical instruments like flutes, lyres, and zithers to heal their patients from illnesses ranging from digestion to mental disturbances and insomnia.

In his famous book De Anima, Aristotle (323–373 BCE) stated that music could purify the mind.

And Egyptians describe how musical incantations could heal sicknesses.

Music has always been present in the life cycle, day and night, and rhythm in all physiological and biological functions is always present.

Modern times research confirms that the music benefits on the body and mind are real, as ancient practitioners described.

So, studies conclude that music can reduce anxiety and stimulate individuals' self-esteem while developing interpersonal skills.

And corresponding to guilt and fear liberation, the 396 hz frequency help to undo traumatic experiences.

While 417, 639, and 741 improve the ability to develop the personality.

Another positive effect of music occurs on the endocrine and anatomic nervous system, greatly reducing recurrent stress.

And results show that when music sounds good to the listener, it soothes and benefits the physiological and hormonal body.

Sound is something powerful and has always impacted people's moods, healing, and well-being.

A modern example is ultrasound which uses high-frequency waves that can detect anomalies in the body through images first used in the 1930s.

And for the 1940s, a doctor in France developed APP or Audio-Psycho -Phonology, a hearing and listening therapy to cure hearing and treat autism and learning.

Coincidentally, Doctor Alfred Tomatis successfully used Gregorian chants in his therapies involving the solfeggio scale.

Today, another doctor, Dr. Horowitz, uses the 528 Hz frequency, the third note in the original Solfeggio, to repair DNA.

At the end of the 16th century, musicians quickly accepted the new creation of twelve-tone equal temperament in Renaissance Italy.

Then the just intonation tuning method using six-tone solfege was gradually used less and eventually replaced.

Besides, David B. Doty, in his book The Just Intonation Primer, comments that the old 6-tone scale had a smoothness and certain clarity that today's 12-tone scale lacks.

Although it is not easy to believe that solfeggio frequencies can cure your diseases by playing some musical notes, we cannot deny the healing effects of music since its effectiveness has a positive confirmation in scientific research.

For example, Greek philosophers like Aristotle and Plato commented on the meaning of music and its beneficial properties.

The Bible and other sources also comment on the positive effects of music.

More recently, in the words of Albert Einstein, we may have been wrong about music because what we call matter is, in fact, energy whose vibration is so low that the senses cannot perceive it.

However, at the correct frequency, sound has a positive effect on your matter, which is your mind and body.

You may have already used calming music to relax your mind or for mental concentration.

However, you may have yet to hear about solfeggio frequencies.

Solfeggio frequencies are sounds that promote overall health for the mind and body.

And studies have confirmed their positive effects in promoting healing and are the same used in Gregorian and Sanskrit chants.

To better understand the importance of solfeggio frequencies, it's essential to consider the Schumann resonance.

In 1952, German physicist Winfried Otto Schumann mathematically recorded the electromagnetic resonances between the Earth's surface and the ionosphere, which is the electrically charged part of the Earth's atmosphere.

Schumann discovered that these electromagnetic waves originated from lightning discharges and resonated at a low frequency between 7.86 Hz to 8 Hz.

He determined that this frequency was equivalent to the Earth's heartbeat and named it the Schumann resonance.

Another physicist, Herbert König, studied this phenomenon and found that these resonances matched levels of human brain activity by comparing EEG recordings with the Earth's electromagnetic field.

These resonances matched five brainwave states: delta, theta, alpha, beta, and gamma.

These states occur daily, from sleeping to creating to learning.

Further research supports König's findings, confirming the integrity of the Schumann resonance and human brain activity.

Other studies indicate that the Schumann resonance synchronizes higher brain function.

And the Solfeggio frequencies have significant positive effects because they resonate harmoniously with the Schumann resonance of 8 Hz.

Musically speaking, the frequencies derive at 8Hz and rise the music scale octave by octave until the C note vibrates at 256 Hz and the A note at 432 Hz.

Tones harmonized with this frequency are known as scientific tuning.

Furthermore, the 432 Hz frequency has particularly beneficial effects.

Music instruments tuned to 432 Hz before the mid-20th century were standard until 440 Hz became common.

And this frequency of 432 Hz is known to be calming and soothing, and its resonance aligns with the Schumann Resonance of 8 Hz.

Recent research indicates that music tuned to 432 Hz slows the heart rate compared to 440 Hz, making it ideal for relaxing activities like yoga, meditation, and sleep.

In 2018, a study from Japan discovered that listening to music tuned to 528 Hz can reduce stress in the nervous system in as little as five minutes.

And the Journal of Addiction Research & Therapy found that 528 Hz can mitigate the toxic effects of ethanol on cells, increasing cell life by up to 20 percent, and its energizing and healing effects make it great for background music or when feeling depressed.

Music tuned to 396 Hz helps to reduce subconscious fears, worries, and anxiety.

And this frequency also eliminates feelings of guilt and negative beliefs that may hinder personal development.

Music can powerfully impact emotions and physical well-being since its frequencies possess unique healing properties.

A 639 Hz frequency. Help regulate emotions encouraging communication, love, and relationships.

The 741 Hz frequency promotes the cleansing of the body and self-expression.

The 852 Hz frequency helps to replace negative thoughts, particularly if you experience nervousness or anxiety.

The Better Sleep app offers these frequencies; you can mix them with other sounds or content, whether working, sleeping, or relaxing.

# Chapter Four

# Injury recovery

"Just like there's always time for pain, there's always time for healing." — Jennifer Brown

Suffering an injury is inevitable since it can occur unexpectedly to everyone.

It can happen when working, playing, resting at home, or on the street.

The human body is a complex and fragile organism.

Prone to bumps and bruises from everyday life.

However, if your injury is not improving, taking the necessary steps to get healthy again is essential.

Finding a recommended physical therapist to aid your recovery is a great decision.

In this regard, you should be aware of some essential steps in the injury recovery process.

**Circumstances:**

The initial circumstances are one of the first things to consider about an accident.

After an accident, the immediate actions taken can drastically impact the recovery process.

Someone who sustains a non-serious injury can decide which action to take.

They may meet with a physical therapist or a doctor for advice on managing their less severe condition. Or the more serious ones.

It's essential to be highly cautious right after sustaining an injury, even when doing basic household tasks.

Due to the possibility of worsening a condition, even when realizing simple tasks at home like making coffee or taking a bath could add to the stress of a shoulder or leg injury.

**The importance of being in repose after an accident is something essential:**

After assessing your injury, the first step is to take it easy and rest the affected area for at least a few days. Avoiding any physical activity during your scheduled time with a physical therapist is vital.

If you are unsure whether your injury is severe and requires treatment, it is advisable to avoid abrupt movements.

Another common yet beneficial practice is applying ice to your injury or some other means available, though ice may not help much in some cases.

**Injury differences:**

Not all injuries are the same. They can vary from sprains, strains, and tears to fractures in arms or legs.

If you experience symptoms of fractures, tears, sprains, or strains, it can be challenging to determine the exact location of the injury.

So, the best step of action is to seek professional medical attention.

A sprain or strain commonly occurs when a ligament or muscle is stretched or pulled.

Generally, in an injury, muscle strain and sprain involve minor tears.

A pulled muscle or strain means that a muscle has suffered a forceful stretching or tearing of a ligament.

Tears are more severe than strains and often happen when the ligament, muscle, or tendon tissue.

rips due to a forceful movement or a brutal hit.

Usually, the injured person may hear or feel a "popping" sensation when the injury occurs.

If the tear is significant, you will experience sudden, severe pain, swelling, and weakness in the affected region.

If the tear is in a joint, it may also result in an inability to flex or extend.

"Fracture, or a broken bone, often will show a deformity in the affected area and an inability to move or bear weight.

If it is an open fracture, there will be an open wound in the injured area."

When there is a significant injury," you should seek immediate urgent care for treatment.

Generally, the injured area may present obvious deformities, inability to move a joint, numbness, weakness, tingling, and often a cold sweat etc.

Some of the most important and known recommendations to treat a strain, tear, or fracture are, for example, the treatment that includes rest, ice, compression, and elevation, which can help mitigate the swelling and pain resulting from an injury.

And stopping any activity will allow the injured area to recover better.

Also, applying an ice pack for 15-20 minutes every two to three hours during the first 48 hours after the injury and covering the ice with a towel to help prevent frostbite is crucial.

Another method to help reduce pain and swelling in minor sprains is compression; however, avoiding tight bandages is essential to prevent numbness in the injured person.

Maintaining the injured area at or above heart level can help heal injured areas of the body, and using folded covers, pillows, or any other object, even something like a stuffed bear, as a sort of elevation for a hurt area is beneficial.

During a medical examination, the first step is to perform an X-ray to evaluate the fracture's severity or the injury's extent.

In case of minor injuries, medical assessments will be cautious and conservative.

Treatment will include R.I.C.E. For rest, ice, compression, elevation, and pain medicine as needed.

The medical specialist will determine the frequency of check-up visits necessary for examination if there are persistent symptoms.

During recovery, the patient may require a splint, crutches, or cane to avoid putting weight on the injured area.

Recovery stages will differ because some people have led their lives differently, taking care of themselves, like their food and way of life.

Also, each person's body has different factors that could affect injury recovery and progression, so having a physical therapist to guide you through your unique case is essential.

The body is complex and requires professional guidance for proper healing.

Recovering from an injury depends on the care you give yourself, as your doctor advises.

It also depends on your effort to get better each day through exercises and other activities that will help you get back in shape as quickly and safely as possible.

The extent of your injury determines the difficulty level of the recovery process.

It can be challenging for anyone who has suffered an injury, but maintaining a positive attitude and being willing to heal is the right approach.

Maintaining contact with your doctor and physical therapist during injury recovery is essential to healing.

Whether or not you are a professional athlete, go slowly in your workouts until your doctor clears you.

When you present these conditions, you can say you have recovered from an injury, including being free from pain and swelling and regaining a complete range of motion in the affected area.

It is more likely for us to ever experience an injury than not.

However, we now understand that we can overcome almost all types of situations, and with the proper assistance, we can progress.

And it is crucial to acknowledge that the human body is fragile, and we must take care of it to prevent injuries or fractures as much as possible."

Here are some essential facts to consider when recovering from a severe injury.

It is vital to understand that recovery may take longer than expected, and patients may feel pressured to return to work before completely recovering.

However, allowing sufficient time for healing and receiving clearance from a doctor before rushing the process is better, as hurrying to heal could delay recovery and worsen the problem.

Of course, there are things a patient can do to help with recovery.

For example, avoid abrupt movements and follow instructions from a physician.

Take the prescribed medicine in the right amount and use the appropriate splint or cane as a doctor directs.

Applying ice, when necessary, can also help reduce swelling and pain.

After recovering from an injury, it is important to continue practicing the exercises that helped you to recover in the first place.

You can even add more exercise if you feel up to it, especially if you are an athlete.

However, it is crucial to be cautious and avoid re-injury.

Always start slowly to warm up and stop exercising if you feel pain or discomfort.

You can resume the exercises once you feel more comfortable or switch to exercises that don't stress the recently recovered injured area of your body.

# Chapter Five

# Healing joints, diet, and exercise

We do not stop exercising because we grow old, we grow old because we stop exercising.

-Dr. Kenneth Cooper

Diet.

Natural healing of joints emphasizes healing without relying on common medications or surgery.

It involves using natural remedies, such as exercise and a diet that helps reduce inflammation.

This approach aims to improve mobility, preventing further damage to joints and muscles.

As we grow older, it's common to experience joint problems.

However, we can take steps to prevent and protect ourselves from joint pain and related issues, enabling us to maintain our daily lives. While some medications can help ease pain, they can create a dependency and have long-term side effects.

Over-the-counter medicines are helpful and can relieve everyday aches and pains and prevent or cure diseases and other health problems ranging from tooth decay to migraines and allergies.

Of course, some alternative medicines can treat muscular and joint aches and pains, as well as

preventing recurring illnesses.

**Gelatin:** For example, Gelatin is an alternative therapy to treat and soothe joints.

Gelatin is an excellent supplement for knee joints, particularly for athletes and sportspeople.

It is a lubricant that prevents bone tissue wear and tear due to regular use.

The protein known as Gelatin comes from the bones and skins of animals and is an ingredient used in various products such as makeup, food, medicines, and vaccines. People with arthritis take gelatin supplements since they contain collagen, a vital component of cartilage that cushions the bones in your joints.

The human body does not absorb collagen precisely by consuming gelatin.

The collagen in gelatin breaks down during digestion, and thus, it does not directly reach the joint areas in the body.

However, there's the belief that gelatin could help alleviate pain in conditions like Osteoarthritis.

A few studies suggest that gelatin helps with some rheumatic arthritis problems in animals. Nevertheless, more reliable information is needed to confirm this.

Ingestion of Gelatin must be under medical supervision, especially when taken in supplements. Although Gelatin is present in various foods and medicines, taking it in supplement form can result in unwanted side effects such as upset stomach, burping, and bloating. Additionally, some people may be prone to allergic reactions due to Gelatin.

The US DEA has stated that consuming Gelatin through food is safe and poses no health risks. However, experts are concerned about the potential dangers of Gelatin supplements, as they may contain animal diseases.

Although there are no reports of disease cases through this means.

It is advisable to consult a doctor before taking Gelatin supplements.

It is also unclear whether Gelatin supplements are safe for children and pregnant or nursing women.

Hydrogel-based scaffolds that transport cells hold great promise in regenerative medicine and could be used to treat conditions such as osteoarthritis.

So, gelatin and glucosamine are the ideal materials to help with cartilage regeneration. However, the weak strength of gelatin hydrogels is a challenge.

To address this, gelatin and glucosamine molecules were grafted with acrylate groups and covalently crosslinked under photo-radiation to form hydrogels.

On the other hand, glucosamine is one of the best supplements for knee joints because its fatty acid is a critical component of cartilage and other joint tissues.

It also helps rebuild bones, prevent cartilage wear, and prevent inflammation of the joints and adjoining muscles.

Supplements that contain glucosamine and chondroitin sulfate can assist in the development of cartilage and prevent joint pain.

Omega-3 Fatty Acids. Help to reduce the wear and tear of the joints. These acids can prevent the enzymes called collagenases from damaging the joints.

These fatty acids help knee joints, reduce inflammation, and strengthen the tendons.

These "healthy fats" support your heart health. And, also significantly, they lower your triglycerides.

Some specific types of omega-3s have properties such as DHA and EPA (found in seafood) and ALA (found in plants).

Some other omega-3 fatty acids are present in foods like salmon, mackerel, flaxseed, and

chia seed.

In simple terms, Omega3s are polyunsaturated fats necessary for your body to perform its functions.

Everybody needs these essential nutrients to survive, and the best way to obtain them is through the foods you eat.

The two primary categories of fatty acids are saturated and unsaturated.

Unsaturated fat further breaks into polyunsaturated and monounsaturated fats, commonly labeled on nutrition products.

Fatty acids are chain-like molecules of carbon, oxygen, and hydrogen atoms.

Carbon atoms form the chain's backbone, while oxygen and hydrogen atoms attach to available slots.

Saturated fat has no more open slots. Monounsaturated fat has one open slot, while polyunsaturated fat has more than one open slot.

Commonly, saturated fats have a relation to increased risk of diseases such as heart and stroke.

Unsaturated (polyunsaturated and monounsaturated) are considered "healthy" fats because they support your heart health, but only if consumed in moderation.

And as a form of polyunsaturated fat, Omega-3s are healthier alternatives to saturated fat.

Tasks of omega-3 fatty acids.

These fatty acids help all the cells in your body function appropriately, and they're a vital part of your cell membranes, which provide structure and support interactions between cells.

While they're essential to cells in the body, omega-3s typically concentrate in high levels in cells, eyes, and brain.

Omega-3s provide energy and support the cardiovascular and endocrine systems.

With its three primary fatty acids,

EPA (eicosatetraenoic acid) is a "marine omega 3" found in fish.

DHA (docosahexaenoic acid) was found in fish.

And alpha-linolenic acid (ALA) is found in plants.

However, these three fatty acids don't provide enough EPA and DHA, so diets with plenty of fish are essential.

Omega-3 fatty acids have potential benefits for cardiovascular health, such as helping to lower triglyceride levels.

Studies show that omega-3s.

Omega-3 fatty acids have potential benefits for cardiovascular health, such as helping to lower triglyceride levels.

When there are too many triglycerides in the blood, the risk of atherosclerosis increases, which can lead to heart disease or stroke.

Therefore, it's essential to keep triglyceride levels under control.

Omega-3s may help lower the risk of developing cardiovascular disease, CVD, abnormal heart rhythm (Arrhythmia, and blood clots.

"Forms of cancer, Alzheimer's, and age-related degeneration are severe health conditions that can significantly affect individuals as they grow older. It is generally better to choose food sources, such as fish, rather than taking pills."

Have regular check-ups of atherosclerotic cardiovascular disease.

High triglycerides (135 to 499 milligrams per Cholesterol under control must be (below 100 mg/dL).

However, Omega-3 benefits are different from regular results.

In some people, the benefits are notable, and in others, not, probably due to variations in the research methods used.

Most kinds of fish add Omega-3 fatty acids to a diet, for example, Mackerel fish, Salmon, Harring, Anchovy, Whitefish, Tuna, Bluefish, Striped bass, and Rainbow trout.

However, other kinds of fish, including King Mackerel, Marlin, Orange rough, Shark, Swordfish, Tilefish, Tuna, Perch, Largemouth bass, striped bass, Pikeminnow, White sturgeon, Blackfish, Catfish, and Black crappie, can carry higher levels of mercury than others.

It is essential to note that consuming too much Fish high in mercury can lead to mercury poisoning and damage your brain, nervous system, and other crucial parts of your organism.

Besides, some people are more sensitive than others to mercury and should avoid it.

Among the groups of people that should avoid Fish with mercury are pregnant women and children under eleven.

For pregnant women and children under eleven, certain kinds of Fish are safe and a source of Omega-3s, but only when eaten in moderation from (ten up to twelve ounces per week)

These types of Fish include. Anchovy, Herring, Mackerel, Salmon, Sardine, Trout, from (freshwater) And Tuna (light, canned)

Albacore, that is (white meat) tuna, has more mercury than canned light tuna.

So, a breastfeeding pregnant woman should eat only six ounces a week.

But to ensure the amounts are safe, the best is to talk with your provider about it.

However, not all people can eat fish because of allergies or a vegetarian style.

Instead, there are options like specific sources of Omega-3 based on plants that provide the nutrients in the form of ALA (Alpha-linolenic acid)

A good source of ALA is milled flaxseed.

And you can easily add it to your meals by sprinkling two tablespoons on your oatmeal, yogurt, or smoothie.

In any case, conversing with your doctor or healthcare provider is the right thing to do.

Algae, canola, chia, edamame, flax, soybean, and walnut oil are sources of ALA.

Safe consumption depends on factors like age.

The recommended quantity of ALA per person varies based on age and other factors.

For example, the recommended amount for men is 1.6 grams.

For women, 1.1 grams.

The recommended daily intake of 1.4 grams is specifically for pregnant women.

Still, the recommendation is to talk with a dietitian.

The American Heart Association recommends consuming at least two servings of fish per week, equivalent to 6 to 8 ounces.

However, if you have a heart disease condition, it is recommended that you consume more foods that contain omega-3 fatty acids.

On the other hand, if you have triglyceride issues, it is better to consult with your doctor before making any dietary changes.

Physical therapy exercises.

Joint problems can be challenging to deal with because they are not as easy to heal as muscles. Joint pains can make it difficult to enjoy simple activities such as walking, going to a park, or doing chores.

These pains can rob you of the joy of performing daily activities you once took for granted.

"Joint pain can impede your ability to carry out daily activities by limiting your range of motion."

This condition can weaken your muscles, leading to increased pain and discomfort.

Moreover, joint pain can interfere with exercises intended to help manage the pain and postpone or avoid surgery.

You can delay surgery and improve your quality of life by performing the right exercises.

You can target joint workouts with a simple walking routine.

First, warm up muscles for better stretching by doing warm-ups before a workout.

Stretch only to mild tension, never to the point of pain, because pain indicates that you are forcing the joints and muscles.

So be careful resetting your initial position and then try again.

It is only a matter of time until flexibility can improve.

When stretching, breathe comfortably and practice it frequently.

Some common joint problems occur in muscles, such as the Achilles tendon, plantar fascia, and other similar body areas.

However, when the problems are related to the Achilles tendon, you can use a towel or other fabric to pull your toes towards your body while keeping your knee straight.

Now, straighten your leg and hold it for 30 seconds on each foot. Repeat three times on each foot.

To perform the plantar fascia, stretch:

Begin by sitting down and resting the arch of your foot on any ball.

Roll your foot over the round object, moving in all directions, for a few minutes.

Aim to repeat this exercise twice a day.

Sitting Plantar Fascia.

For this exercise, sit down and cross one foot over your knee to perform the Sitting Plantar Fascia stretch.

Start by grasping the base of your toes and pulling them back towards your body until you feel a comfortable stretch.

Hold this position for 15-20 seconds.

Hold onto the base of your toes and gently pull them towards your body. Stop when you feel comfortable stretching.

Stretch, and then release. Repeat this process three times to complete the exercise.

Wall push is a standard exercise that helps to improve mobility by stretching. Follow these steps to perform the exercise:

1. Stand facing a wall.

2. Place both hands on the wall at shoulder height.

3. Put one foot in front of the other, with the front foot around 30cm (12 inches) from the wall.

4. Bend the front knee towards the wall while keeping the back knee straight.

5. Stop when the calf in your back leg feels tight.

6. Relax and repeat the process ten times.

Next, repeat the first step and move the back foot forward slightly while slightly bending the back knee. Repeat this process ten times.

Ankle range of motion is another specific exercise in which you Bend your ankle up towards your body, then point your toes away. Repeat ten times.

Ankle rotation.

In this exercise, slowly move your ankle in a circular motion. Repeat this ten times in each direction.

For the "Towel Pickup" exercise, please follow these steps:

1. Sit on a chair with a towel in front of you.

2. Keep your heel firmly on the ground and use your toes to scrunch up the towel.

3. Repeat this motion 10 to 20 times.

4. As you improve, you can add a small weight to the towel (such as a tin of beans) to increase the difficulty of the exercise.

Stand heel raise.

You can use a chair, a wall, or a counter for support to perform a standing heel raise. Keep your knees straight and rise on your tiptoes. Hold the position for about 3 seconds, then slowly lower your feet. Repeat this exercise around ten times.

Toe spread.

While sitting on a chair, take one of your feet and place your fingers between each toe.

Hold onto your heel and rotate your foot for ten rotations, holding your ankle with the other hand. Then, reverse the direction.

You can bend and flex your foot to help with stiffness and pain.

Writing in alphabet writing is an excellent exercise for foot and ankle strength.

While sitting on a chair or the floor, try writing the alphabet, pointing your big toe in the air, and moving just your ankle. Write the whole alphabet at least once a day.

Ankle out.

To perform this exercise, you will need a piece of elastic band to form a loop.

Fix the loop to a table leg or secure it under your opposite foot.

Place one foot in the loop and turn your toes outwards, feeling the band's resistance.

Gradually bring your foot back to its initial position.

Repeat this exercise twice a day.

Physical exercise.

It is optional to have specialized equipment available to start exercising.

Today, various apps, videos, and other resources are available to help you get started with physical exercise.

"When exercising, wearing comfortable clothing and appropriate sports footwear is essential.

It doesn't have to be expensive, but it should be suitable for the type of physical exercise you are doing.

Wearing comfortable shoes is especially important as they provide support to help absorb any shock and protect your joints and muscles from the strenuous efforts during exercise."

When frequently exercising, staying hydrated by drinking enough water for general well-being is crucial.

Warm-up before starting a workout session is the best way to prepare the body for increased efforts and reduce the risk of injury.

Warming also helps increase the heart rate and temperature in the muscles so they are ready for physical exercise.

Some examples of warming up include jogging, jumping, walking, and stretching to the point of being slightly short of breath.

Similarly, it is necessary to cool down after exercising so that the heart rate and muscles can return to a state of relaxation and calmness.

It is essential to understand that regular exercise is the best way to maintain good health and a positive outlook.

Start slowly and gradually build the intensity to help the body avoid experiencing pain during the activity.

So, you can enjoy the effort and the benefits of a complete connection between the mind and body.

Having a personal doctor or a physiotherapist is only sometimes necessary to get started with exercise.

However, the best is to start slowly without worrying or trying to work out in excess.

But if you need to ask your physician or fitness instructor, it is also correct.

If you have some condition or need to work on specific exercises, ask for help from a professional trainer or physiotherapist.

# Chapter 6

# Wellness through plants

"We might think we are nurturing our garden, but of course it's our garden that is really nurturing us."

– Jenny Uglow

Powerful health benefits of plants.

Plants add life to any space, whether in a garden or indoors.

"And not only can they make a place look better, but they can also confer a sense of coziness and well-being just by being around them.

Not to mention the many more benefits they bring to people's lives."

The human immune system is capable of fighting viruses on its own.

This capability of fighting foreign threats creates a safe environment for the human body to rest and develop properly, allowing for a more robust immune system.

When surrounded by plants, the human body can benefit from chemicals released, boosting the immune system, and helping fight illness.

Therefore, people who keep indoor plants can naturally repel bugs and experience fewer headaches, skin issues, and even nausea.

In other words, plants are powerful invisible healers, whether they are intended for decoration or not.

Excellent properties of houseplants.

Plants possess some remarkable qualities that make them excellent air purifiers. They can filter harmful toxins from the air, creating a healthier living environment. In addition to improving air quality, they also provide other benefits that promote overall well-being.

Aloe Vera.

One of the plants worth considering is Aloe Vera.

This plant grows exceptionally well indoors and offers numerous benefits.

Aloe Vera can be used in juices or applied topically to the skin. To ensure its proper growth, keep the plant in a warm area where it can receive natural light. Avoid overwatering.

Spider Plants.

Like several other plants, Spider Plants can purify the air by removing carbon monoxide, benzene, formaldehyde, and other pollutants.

This plant enhances the oxygen levels in a room and improves human body functions.

Spider plants can quickly grow indoors in the proper condition and thrive in indirect light.

These plants require frequent watering during the summer, but they do not need to be watered during winter.

Snake Plants.

Snake Plants are one of the most accessible plants to care for.

Snake plants can decrease the pollutants commonly found in household products, making them an excellent choice for indoor environments.

In addition, these plants help with sleep, making them ideal for placement in bedrooms.

These plants are resistant and can thrive in reduced water and light conditions.

It's best to provide indirect light and only water them when the soil is dry.

Chrysanthemums not only add beauty to the surroundings, but they also have a positive impact on our health.

Chrysanthemums help to improve people's well-being by removing benzene from the air.

Additionally, these plants are suitable for making teas, which have various health benefits.

However, taking care of chrysanthemums may require more effort than taking care of other plants.

These plants need direct sunlight, warmer temperatures, and water more often to thrive.

Warneck Dracaenas

Dracaenas are excellent air purifiers that can help alleviate allergies and asthma symptoms. They are low-maintenance plants that thrive in filtered light. Being adapted to low light, they require less water, but it's still essential to keep their soil and leaves moist.

Other immune-boosting properties of Warneck Dracaenas include:

Reducing stress and anxiety.

Absorbing odors and molds.

Giving headache relief.

Improving mood.

Improving brain function.

Increasing energy levels.

Boosting healing.

Lowering blood pressure.

Plants are not only great for reducing stress levels, but they can also help people concentrate on their work and reduce fatigue while improving focus. Therefore, adding some plants to your workspace can be very beneficial. Peace lilies, philodendron, and lemon balm are some of the best plants to keep in a workspace.

Plants are well known for purifying the air by removing toxins and pollutants.

In countries like Australia, where people spend significant time indoors, plants are considered essential for daily life.

When suffering from headaches, fatigue, or nausea due to poor air quality? Adding beneficial plants can help alleviate these discomforts.

Plants like English ivy, spider plants, and Chinese evergreens can reduce indoor air pollution.

Indoor plants cannot only decorate the halls and rooms of hospitals due to their many benefits but also have the potential to promote and even create sensations of happiness by releasing the oxygen that people need to boost their health.

In addition, taking care of plants can add a sense of accomplishment, making anyone feel better. Plants like Lavender, Jasmine, and Aloe Vera are also vital to boost people's mental health and experience sensations of well-being.

Plants are great at fighting air pollution by filtering out pollen, dust, and mold since plants are natural air purifiers that work effectively to eliminate air pollutants.

You can benefit from indoor plants like Peace Lily, bamboo, and Janet Craig plants if you have allergies.

However, it's best to avoid Daisies and Sunflowers if you have allergies.

Indoor plants offer several benefits to humans, including reducing stress levels.

Stress can negatively impact your natural ability to sleep, affecting your overall well-being. Additionally, the scent of certain plants can have therapeutic qualities that can help you fall asleep more easily.

Lavender, jasmine, and gardenia are the best aromatic plants for relaxation and sleep.

Besides, research has shown that plants can positively influence our well-being, making us happier and healthier.

According to Libby Bolles from Fancy Leaf Plant Co. in Parrish, Florida, caring for plants can bring health and wellness into our lives.

So, who would want to avoid feeling healthy and enjoying the benefits of plants?

According to researchers, Plants have various health benefits, including improving concentration for students and office workers.

Many office buildings and hospitals decorate their spaces with plants.

And the reason to have many indoor plants is because these plants offer many and diverse benefits.

Certain emotions arise when seeing plants, green grass, or many trees.

It is a feeling that can be compared to coming home after a long absence.

We feel comfortable when we are near plants because plants have a calming effect on our nerves and can help reduce anxiety.

Once you have discovered the advantages of having plants, you must learn how to take care of them properly and identify the best ones that suit your needs.

It is advisable to consult with an expert from a local garden shop to get started on your plant-growing journey.

When owning plants, consider choosing resilient options like Snake Plants that are hard to kill.

Orchids. They require more care, but they are worth having at home or the office; their scent is fragrant and beautiful to watch.

Spider plants. With their cascading leaves, they adapt quickly everywhere.

Peperomia plants. With their oval fleshy leaves, they tend to look for sun rays.

Jade plants are succulent and can grow extensively but can be easily pruned and shaped.

Caring for plants is an art that can be challenging but ultimately rewarding.

# Chapter 7

# Defying aging

It's not how old you are, it's how you are old.

— Jules Renard

There is no apparent cause or reason why we age.

Researchers have tried to understand the mechanisms that take place on mutations in chromosomes, mitochondria, junk inside and outside cells, and the link between proteins and aging.

Additionally, there is a phenomenon where, after a certain age, the cells in the body no longer divide but do not die, which could allow other cells to divide.

Scientists are now discussing two theories on why we age.

Some theorize that aging occurs because of a loss of stem cell availability, while others maintain that we are aging due to our usefulness for reproductive purposes as we get old.

To enhance longevity, we must understand the mechanisms that enable optimal human body function and the factors contributing to aging.

There is the knowledge that the accumulation of metabolic waste, which the body can no longer break down, and the failure of biological systems contribute to increased cellular damage, affecting every organ, and causing rapid aging.

How aging processes in the molecules affect the biological systems of the body.

The skeletal system: Specifically in men, bone density diminishes around age thirty-five, and the process starts earlier in women.

In postmenopausal women, the rate of bone loss accelerates. As the discs between the vertebrae in the spine lose fluid, it speeds up the process of losing height. Additionally, mineral loss causes the long bones in the body to become brittle, and the joints become stiffer and less flexible as they lose their fluid.

Less fluid causes the cartilage to rub together, wearing out and leading to the deposition of minerals in and around the joints.

As we age, both men and women tend to experience a decline in their skeletal muscle mass. This condition is known as Sarcopenia, which can worsen in the absence of triggers such as regular exercise.

This gradual muscle loss can lead to decreased strength, flexibility, coordination, balance, and height.

The deterioration of the central nervous system can hinder the ability to recruit muscle fibers, and this loss leads to poor posture and a greater risk of bone fractures, which can cause inflammation, pain, stiffness, and even physical deformities.

Engaging in regular physical activity that involves stretching the muscles and the skeletal system can help slow down the aging process.

The digestive system: Also, our digestive system tends to slow down gradually.

The muscles that contract and push food along the digestive tract also slow down, causing waste to move slowly through the colon.

The slower the waste moves, the more water it loses, which worsens constipation.

Moreover, lower physical activity in older people contributes to even :more significant problems.

As we grow older, our body's capacity to generate natural digestive enzymes declines, which can reduce protein absorption.

This enzyme deficiency can worsen sarcopenia by losing muscle mass and strength.

Enzymes are vital in building, integrating, transporting, providing, and eliminating various nutrients and toxins.

Our body's capacity to generate natural digestive enzymes declines as we age.

Respiratory system: As we age, our respiratory system starts to decline. After age 25, if a person is not exercising regularly, their lung capacity and maximum oxygen utilization (V02 max) decrease gradually.

The respiratory muscles weaken, and the effectiveness of the lung's defense mechanism decreases, including a reduction in the quantity of white blood cells on the surface of the lung alveoli.

As we age, the alveoli lose shape and starts to function poorly.

Even changes in the spine and ribs can affect the respiratory system's effectiveness, and the part of the brain that controls breathing can reduce lung capacity, negatively affecting overall health in various ways.

However, regular cardiovascular exercise can help maintain the respiratory system's health.

Urinary system: As we grow older, between the ages of thirty and forty, our kidneys experience a gradual decline in their filtering rate, and it happens because the kidneys lose tissue, and the filter units, called nephrons, decrease in number.

Additionally, the bladder wall loses its elasticity, making it difficult to hold as much urine as before, and the muscles that control the bladder also weaken.

Also, the urethra becomes blocked by an enlarged prostate gland in men or by a prolapsed or fallen bladder or vagina in women.

Staying adequately hydrated and maintaining a balanced mineral intake is essential to control these issues.

A recommendation is to limit the consumption of dehydrating substances such as alcohol and caffeine while avoiding excess protein.

Reproductive system: Women typically experience menopause around the age of 51. And the ovaries, which produce hormones such as estrogen and progesterone, stop functioning and no longer produce eggs.

As a result, women can no longer conceive after menopause.

However, the risk of developing a yeast infection increases, and the external genital and breast tissue may become thinner.

Men do not experience a significant change in fertility with age, but testicular tissue mass, testosterone, and blood flow to the reproductive organs gradually decline.

Endocrine system: The hypothalamus, a part of the brain, produces hormones that control other structures in the endocrine system.

Although the levels of these regulating hormones remain the same while you age, the response of other endocrine organs to those hormones may diminish.

Human growth hormone begins to decline at a rate of fourteen percent per decade in both men and women starting at the age of thirty.

When women go through menopause, their levels of progesterone, testosterone, and estrogen begin to fall.

At the age of fifty, thyroid activity starts to decrease, and it may lead to hyper or hypothyroidism.

As people reach fifty years of age, they may experience a reduction in the production of a hormone called DHEA (dehydroepiandrosterone), which puts people at risk for types of cancer.

Moreover, when people reach sixty, their insulin production decreases, and insulin cell receptors become less sensitive, which impairs the body's ability to metabolize sugar, which increases the risk of diabetes.

At the age of seventy, there is a decline in the hormones that protect against calcium loss.

This loss of calcium makes the human body more susceptible to osteoporosis.

The natural hormone replacement industry is experiencing a boom as it helps alleviate endocrine issues arising with age.

However, traditional practices such as consuming organic meat, engaging in regular sexual activity, and avoiding endocrine-disrupting chemicals in food can still be effective alternatives.

Circulatory system: The circulatory system changes at forty when the heart muscles and blood vessels thicken, causing the heart to fill with blood more slowly.

However, athletes who practice lifting or other hard practicing sports may experience this problem with blood occurring earlier in their lives due to the heart pumping harder to carry blood to the vessels.

High blood pressure and other cardiovascular problems, such as arrhythmias, may also make people experience dizziness when standing up from a chair or after lying down because of exacerbated cardiovascular issues.

Such issues as calcium deposits in the body can cause stiffening of joints, plaque buildup on the teeth, a hardening of arteries, impaired brain functions, and general aches or pain.

After the age of sixty, people tend to have enlarged calcium deposits in their arteries, often caused by a lack of minerals in the diet, dehydration, limescale in tap water, or synthetic calcium consumption in supplements.

As we age, we can experience abnormal heart rhythms, commonly known as arrhythmias. Atrial fibrillation is one such condition that can develop after the age of sixty. The heart's natural pacemaker, responsible for regulating the heartbeat rate, can also be affected by age-related issues. Some of its pathways may develop fibrous tissue and fat deposits, resulting in a slower heart rate due to the loss of some of its cells.

The lymphatic fluid circulating through the body is a part of the circulatory system.

After the age of forty, these lymphatic fluids can stagnate, causing toxins to accumulate and weakening the immune system, making it difficult to fight infections and diseases.

However, regular exercise, hydration, and exposure to heat and cold can help maintain good health.

To reinforce the immune system, take vitamins such as vitamin C.

And plant-based foods are the best natural source of vitamin C.

Fruits such as oranges, grapefruits, limes, and lemons contain high amounts of vitamin C.

Still, other non-citrus fruits like papayas, strawberries, pineapples, kiwis, cantaloupes, and raspberries are also rich in this essential vitamin.

One of the most crucial habits to adopt is quitting smoking or avoiding it altogether to improve your chances of living a long and healthy life.

However, there is something that we can do to undo the damage of smoking.

The main downsides of smoking include the following.

Formation of habits is a common occurrence when one becomes addicted to nicotine due to its impact on the central nervous system.

Withdrawal symptoms, such as anxiety, irritability, depression, headaches, and sleep problems, may arise when attempting to quit smoking. Emphysema is when the air sacs in the lungs are irreversibly damaged.

Lung cancer is also a potential risk.

The constriction and damage of blood vessels due to smoking can lead to peripheral artery disease and hypertension, a chronic condition characterized by elevated blood pressure. Furthermore, smoking increases the risk of stroke.

A plant-based diet uses a small amount of animal protein as a staple food from plants or animals.

Traditional staples such as legumes and grains like quinoa, amaranth, and millet are essential to many cultures' diets.

Millet is a fast-growing cereal plant widely known in warm countries and regions with poor soil in central Africa.

The numerous tiny millet seeds are great for making flour or alcoholic drinks.

The recommendation is also to consume sweet potatoes and corn tortillas.

Avoid processed and packaged food.

Many common foods perceived as healthy and found in the "healthy food" section of supermarkets, convenience stores, and airport newsstands actually contain harmful ingredients. These foods include refined carbohydrates, artificial flavors, processed vegetable oils, and natural sweeteners. Some examples are packaged dried fruits, trail mix, and energy bars. These items often contain blood-sugar-spiking or inflammation-producing compounds, such as simple carbohydrates and vegetable oils, deceptively labeled as organic sunflower oil, cane sugar, or agave syrup.

It's essential to be aware of these ingredients and read labels carefully to make informed decisions about what you eat.

Eat legumes.

A legume is a dry food contained within the shell or pod of a plant, and the most known are beans, peas, peanuts, lentils, garbanzo, and alfalfa.

Legumes are rich in plant protein, vitamins, minerals, appetite-satiating, and gut-supporting fiber.

It is unclear whether the longevity gained from legume consumption is because of the inclusion of slow-release carbohydrates such as white flour or whether the nutrient density of legumes is what makes them so unique.

"Please remember the following: 'Remain reproductively useful."

It's essential to remain reproductively helpful to optimize longevity.

In other words, staying useful means that you should consistently send your body and brain the message that you are a valuable, contributing member of society, especially when it comes to the propagation of your species.

To achieve this, you should avoid retiring, continue learning new things, and avoid surrounding yourself with older, sedentary people in nursing homes or hospice settings.

Instead, continue to have sex, have children, or both to stay active and engaged.

Research conducted in laboratories suggests that regular sex and childbearing have benefits that support the idea that aging is not a programmed death process selected for the good of the species. Instead, aging occurs because natural selection is weak and ineffective at maintaining survival, reproduction, and cellular repair.

As we age, our bodies experience deterioration that is detrimental to reproductive success and shortens our lifespan.

However, longevity may still show more adverse effects when our reproductive events decrease.

In the book "Does Aging Stop?", Dr. Michael Rose suggests that aging can plateau or stop in later stages of life.

He points to demographic data from his large-scale fruit fly experiments and data on humans, both of which support the hypothesis that acceleration in death rates can halt in later life.

Rose had several suggestions for improving this plateau.

One of his more effective tips was to have many children and a happy married life early on, then continue having children as late as possible while leading an active lifestyle even in old age.

Although controversial, he believed reducing grain and agriculture consumption could slow down age-related damage.

There is a fascinating story about a Chinese man named Li Ching-Yuen, who reportedly lived to be 256 years old.

\He was said to be a well-loved figure in his community, having been married 23 times and fathering over 200 children.

If Yuen's story is true, he may be the best example that maintaining reproductive health with age could be an excellent idea.

Most people who live long, healthy, and happy lives have found ways to incorporate low-level physical activity throughout their day by modifying their environment.

Instead of being sedentary most of the day and then doing intense exercise at the start or end of the day, they keep moving all day long.

Exercising during most of the day can be achieved through various ways, such as keeping a pull-up bar or kettlebell at their workplace, taking frequent walks, or using treadmill workstations.

Therefore, this week, try to change your environment to enable more movement by, for instance, only sitting or lying down when necessary, such as while eating or driving.

# Chapter 8

# Lean and mean.

Those who don't jump will never fly.

-Leena Ahmad Almashat

However, this notion is only partially true since it violates the law of conservation of mass, which states that mass cannot be created nor destroyed in an isolated system. Contrary to popular belief, fat is not pooped out or turned into muscle either. Interestingly, fat is primarily excreted through your lungs when you lose weight.

When it comes to losing weight, many believe that fat is converted into energy or heat, as weight-loss experts, physicians, dietitians, and personal trainers suggested.

However, this is only partially true and goes against the law of conservation of mass, which states that mass is not created nor destroyed in an isolated system.

Contrary to popular belief, fat is not pooped out or turned into muscle. Instead, the excess carbohydrates or protein you consume, including the half-stick of butter you may add to your coffee, are transformed into triglycerides, and stored in fat cells.

Additionally, extra dietary fat undergoes lipolysis, which is the breakdown of fat, followed by re-esterification to store mass in adipocytes.

Interestingly, fat is primarily excreted through your lungs when you lose weight.

People who want to lose weight while maintaining their muscles and other vital tissues aim to burn through the triglycerides stored in adipocytes.

Triglycerides contain carbon, hydrogen, and oxygen atoms and can only disappear through oxidation, which requires oxygen.

When you struggle to lose weight, simply dieting or exercising may not be the solution.

Even if you exercise often, it is time to consider other factors preventing you from achieving your weight loss goals.

According to research, strength training can improve your ability to transport glucose into your muscles.

Strength training can lower blood glucose levels and increase insulin sensitivity, even lifting only 30 percent of your single-repetition maximum weight (IRM).

IRM refers to controlling blood sugar, upregulating sugar transporters, and reducing sugar storage as fat with relatively light bodyweight exercises like push-ups, air squats, and lunges.

When done correctly, the Incomplete Rest Method (IRM) is a quick and efficient way to create a metabolic stimulus with minimal inflammation or mechanical damage.

It is beneficial for achieving body composition goals and has various other applications.

According to research, exercising before breakfast, especially in a fasted state, is a powerful approach to managing blood sugar levels.

An Ayurvedic technique described in books such as Suhas Kshirsagar states that a "Change of Schedule can also Change Your Life."

In one study, participants were told to exercise before eating, drink only water during training, and then eat a large breakfast afterward. Despite consuming a large breakfast, the group participants gained almost no weight, and their metabolic rates increased.

As a result, they burned the energy they consumed later in the day more efficiently.

So, the recommendation is to get some exercise before eating your gluten-free muffin or smoothie or take a handful of fish oil pills.

After a meal, walking is more effective than standing; therefore, standing is better than sitting.

One study showed that standing for 180 minutes after lunch reduced post-lunch blood sugar spikes by 43 percent.

Another study found that alternating between standing and sitting every thirty minutes throughout the workday reduced blood sugar spikes by 11.1 percent on average.

So, even during a day at the office, you don't have to work out to control your blood sugar.

The trick is to only sit down for part of your workday and to hack your office environment, so you stay physically active all day long.

If you find yourself in situations where you are unable to exercise, must sit for long hours at work, or are on a long flight, you can still manage your blood sugar levels by consuming certain plants, herbs, and spices. Some effective spices include Ceylon cinnamon, Gymnema Sylvestre, berberine, rock lotus (shilianhua or stone lotus), and bitter melon extract.

These natural ingredients and compounds can help prevent diabetes by reducing the duration and intensity of blood glucose spikes.

Insulin functions: Insulin is critical in protein metabolism in muscle tissue and has both anabolic and anticatabolic effects.

Insulin metabolism is essential for muscle growth and repair because it facilitates the transport of amino acids into muscle tissue, making them available for muscle protein synthesis.

Additionally, insulin helps reduce muscle protein breakdown.

Thyroid function: The hormone thyroxine (T4) is produced in the thyroid gland and then converted into the more active hormone triiodothyronine (T3).

The upregulated hormone conversion by insulin significantly decreases during excessive caloric or carbohydrate restriction periods.

Bone health: Osteoblasts secrete hydroxyapatite crystals to create new bone tissue and remineralize existing bone matrix.

Insulin increases osteoblast activity, proliferation, differentiation, and survival while enhancing connective tissue integrity.

Healthy immune responses: When insulin elevates, immune cells become more stable.

Insulin activates immune cells called neutrophils.

(the first line of defense during infection or injury) and other immune system sentinel cells.

It even enhances the effectiveness of natural killer cells, which destroy infected cancerous cells.

It also activates helper T cells, which assist with immune attacks, and regulatory T cells, which modulate immune responses and prevent autoimmune diseases.

High insulin levels can cause inflammation by promoting the spread and movement of regulatory T cells.

At the same time, autoimmune problems and immune system suppression relate to insulin resistance or consistently low insulin levels. Therefore, blocking insulin can decrease the growth and movement of regulatory T cells, and high insulin levels can be inflammatory.

Central nervous system:

Insulin can pass through the blood-brain barrier and attach to receptors in various brain areas.

It can attach to receptors in the hypothalamus and hippocampus region, which helps to decrease hunger and regulate energy levels. Additionally, it can enhance cognitive functions such as neuroplasticity, learning, and memory.

Poor insulin signaling in the brain is related to cognitive impairment, dementia, and Alzheimer's disease.

Insulin protects our brain against inflammation by binding to receptors on microglial cells, the brain's resident immune cells.

When insulin levels are low in the brain, it increases the level of inflammatory cytokines in neural tissue. Intranasal insulin can treat this insulin deficiency in individuals with deficient insulin levels.

Hormone regulation: Insulin works in conjunction with insulin-like growth factor 1 and follicle-stimulating hormone to increase the production of estrogen and testosterone in the body.

Insulin also reduces the levels of sex hormone-binding globulin in the blood, which is responsible for binding to testosterone and estrogen and making them inactive, meaning that, up to a certain point, higher levels of insulin can boost the production of sex hormones and improve their bioavailability.

Insulin also interacts with cortisol, growth hormone, glucagon, and other neurotransmitters such as dopamine, serotonin, and melatonin.

Cortisol and stress: When you feel stressed, your body releases hormones like cortisol.

These hormones activate functions necessary for immediate survival, such as higher blood pressure and quick decision-making.

Meanwhile, cortisol suppresses nonessential functions like immune function, digestion, and protein synthesis, a process helpful if you need to handle an acute stressor.

However, cortisol also has a downside.

It suppresses insulin secretion, inhibits glucose uptake into your cells, and disrupts insulin signaling to muscle tissue.

Then chronic stress can cause insulin resistance, leading to weight-loss resistance, inflammation, dyslipidemia (elevated blood fat and cholesterol levels), and hypertension.

The assumption is that several factors can cause a spike in cortisol, a stress hormone.

These factors include the death of a loved one, losing a job, academic stress, and experiencing negative emotions such as boredom, anger, depression, fear, and anxiety.

Toxins and pollutants in your food or environment, high altitude, poor oxygen availability, constant attention from social media, and lack of encouragement or love from others are also stressors that can cause a spike in cortisol.

One way to determine if you are chronically stressed is to monitor your heart rate variability (HRV). HRV refers to the variability in the time between each heartbeat and can be used to assess your nervous system's health status.

When the nerves arising from the brain and the spinal cord that supply the internal organs and blood vessels activate, they release acetylcholine, which induces a low heart rate and relaxation.

At this point, HRV is typically at its highest, indicating a low state of stress.

If you're not well-rested, your heart's beat-to-beat variation can decrease, indicating a severe stress issue if you consistently have low HRV values.

Sleep deprivation: A lack of sleep is unfavorable to your body.

It can increase cortisol levels, reduce glucose tolerance, and increase sympathetic nervous system activity.

Research has found that lack of sleep can decrease insulin sensitivity and glucose tolerance. This lack of sleep leads to lower levels of the hormone leptin, which stimulates feelings of fullness, allowing the hormone ghrelin, which increases hunger, to be more prevalent.

This combination can make you crave sugary and unhealthy snacks, leading to overeating. Therefore, when you're sleep-deprived, reaching for a second helping or giving in to vending machine snacks is expected.

Snacking and post-workout calories: The theory that eating small meals during the day is necessary to keep your metabolism high is a wrong assumption that is now widely known.

While digestion does produce a thermic effect that increases metabolism, the bump is minor.

Frequent snacking can increase the variability of your blood sugar levels and prevent you from reaping the gut and longevity-boosting benefits of fasting. It also forces your metabolism to rely on sugar for fuel instead of tapping into the fat stored in your body.

However, no evidence suggests that eating more than three meals daily can boost your metabolism, help you lose weight, or control your appetite.

In contrast, if you limit your eating to three meals a day within a compressed eating window, your body will burn fat and release more anti-aging and growth hormones, meaning that consuming six small meals per day may be more detrimental to your waistline than consuming two or three larger meals spread throughout the day.

The belief that not eating more during the day leads to starvation is untrue.

Only after more than three days of fasting can the body start downregulating metabolism and thyroid processes.

Research has shown that short-term fasts, such as daily overnight twelve- to sixteen-hour fasts, can increase your metabolic rate by signaling fat cells to break down due to increased norepinephrine, one of the hormones.

However, you don't have to reduce your caloric intake, especially if you are active.

Instead, the key is to eat less often, not to eat less.

Not moving enough: Remember to take frequent breaks every twenty-five to fifty minutes, whether standing, lunging, kneeling, sitting, or leaning.

During these breaks, engage in kettlebell swings, quick strolls up the stairs, jumping jacks, or a handful of burpees. You can even pull over during long road trips to do a hundred jumping jacks for each hour of driving and do forty air squats in a restaurant stall; it's worth checking if you can perform elaborate stretch routines at the back of airplanes. Etc.

To lose weight, you need to burn more calories than you consume through your diet.

So, instead of being an exercise addict, focus on creating an energy deficit through physical activity and a healthy diet.

Excessive sitting for eight hours a day can harm your health, regardless of whether you exercise regularly.

Exercising more is necessary to prevent the adverse effects of a sedentary lifestyle.

If you don't, you may be at a higher risk of developing metabolic syndrome, obesity, type 2 diabetes, cardiovascular disease, and premature mortality.

Therefore, it's crucial to be aware of how much time you spend sitting and make an effort to move around more frequently throughout the day.

Extended periods of regular inactivity can cause your blood sugar levels to become unstable because of insufficient physical activity.

They can lead to adverse changes in insulin signaling, glucose transport, and lipoprotein lipase activity.

The solution is to be more active at work when people tend to move the least.

We discussed different factors that can prevent you from losing weight and how to reverse those effects to get the desired body.

But before attaining a perfect shredded body, you should first understand that everybody is different, and so is everybody,

Your body may have reached its ideal weight even if you are unsatisfied with your physique according to the beauty standards of magazines and pop culture.

Your body may have already reached a healthy balance, even if you have a higher-than-desired body fat percentage. It may not seem fair, but it's the truth.

"If you're following a healthy diet and exercise routine but still not losing weight, it's possible that your body has reached a stable state where it's genetically not inclined to have visible veins in your abs, striated lats, or skinny calves.

However, it's essential to understand that this is perfectly normal and acceptable."

Trying to lose weight with excessive exercise and dieting with an orthorexic approach while pushing your body to its limits with fat-loss biohacks is not the way to go.

This approach is more likely to downregulate your overall well-being, such as relationships, satisfaction, and happiness.

Instead, accept the fact that you have a unique body.

At the same time, you work, take cold showers, avoid sitting for long periods, practice deep diaphragmatic breathing, implement intermittent fasting, and use other unconventional fat-loss techniques to enhance fat loss and your overall health.

Remember to appreciate and enjoy your body for what it is.

# Thank You

Thank you for reading this book.

Please take a moment to write a review, it helps more than you know.

Your feedback is instrumental in helping me grow as a writer and reach others who may benefit from these ideas. Would you consider leaving a review on your favorite online bookstore? Every honest review, whether short or long, positive or constructive, helps me understand how this book has impacted you and provides valuable insights for future readers.

Think of it as paying it forward – your review can help others discover this message and embark on their own transformation. Whether you share your favorite takeaways, highlight specific chapters that resonated, or offer suggestions for improvement, your voice matters.

Thank you again for being a part of this journey. I believe in the power of sharing knowledge and hope this book continues to inspire you long after you finish the last sentence.

With sincere gratitude,

A. Gabriel

# Don't miss out!

Visit the website below and you can sign up to receive emails whenever A. Gabriel publishes a new book. There's no charge and no obligation.

https://books2read.com/r/B-A-MLHDB-SSHVC

**BOOKS 2 READ**

Connecting independent readers to independent writers.

# Also by A. Gabriel

Health improvement through Body Knowledge